Shiatsu
Japanese Healing Massage
for Relaxation and Well-being

Copyright © 1998 Könemann Verlagsgesellschaft mbH
Bonner Str. 126, D-50968 Cologne

Realization: Könemann Verlagsgesellschaft mbH
Editor: KVM Dr. Kolster und Co. Produktions- und
Verlags-GmbH, Marburg
Photography: Lutz Pape
Editor: Dr. Sabine Klapp
Layout: LOGO
Graphic Design: Matthias Grabowski
Cover Design: Peter Feierabend, Steffi Weischer

Original title: Shiatsu. Entspannung und Wohlbefinden durch japanische Heilmassage

Copyright © 1999 for the English edition
Könemann Verlagsgesellschaft mbH

Managing Editor: Bettina Kaufmann
Project Management: Kristin Zeier
Translation from German: Susan Bennett
Editor of the English-language Edition: Lynn Brown in association with Goodfellow & Egan, Cambridge
Typesetting: Goodfellow and Egan, Cambridge
Project Manager for Goodfellow & Egan: Jackie Dobbyne
Production Manager: Detlev Schaper
Assistants: Nicola Leurs, Alexandra Kiesling
Printing and Binding: Sing Cheong Printing Co. Ltd., Hong Kong

Printed in Hong Kong, China

ISBN 3-8290-2011-2

10 9 8 7 6 5 4 3 2 1

Shiatsu

Japanese Healing Massage
for Relaxation and Well-being

Dr. Bernard Kolster

A Far-Eastern Healing Method

Activating powers of self-healing
Relaxation and tranquillity
Step-by-step instructions
Massage yourself or a partner

KÖNEMANN

Summary of video contents

Contents

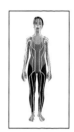

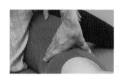

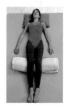

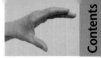

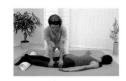

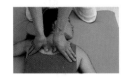

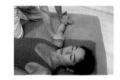

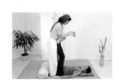

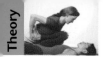

Foreword

The fascinating world of Shiatsu

I first came across Shiatsu a few years ago and soon became fascinated with this extraordinary method of healing. In order to understand Shiatsu, one must first get to grips with the difference between the medicine of the Far East and that of the west.

In our western world medicine is, by and large, symptom-oriented, i.e. treatment is generally directed at the individual parts of the body that are affected, whereas the eastern point of view sees the person fundamentally as a whole. Health depends not upon the "functioning" of parts of the body, but upon the undisturbed flow and harmonious distribution of vital energy in the total organism. According to this point of view, illnesses generally arise from an imbalance in the distribution of this energy. Consequently, an important foundation of the eastern art of healing is the recognition and treatment of imbalances of energy in the body. The treatments employed for this purpose can be divided into several groups: massage, acupressure, acupuncture, breathing therapy, meditation, diet and medication (chiefly herbal in origin). These number among the important components of eastern medicine, a group to which Shiatsu also belongs.

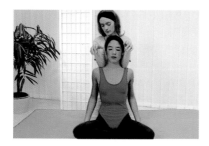

Obviously it is only possible to scratch the surface of this multi-faceted theme in a practical guide such as this which is designed to serve as an introduction to Shiatsu, with a firm emphasis on its practical application. Shiatsu is best

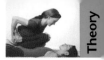

experienced through one's own body, and I have selected just a few of the main techniques and modified them so that they are easy to do. My aim has been to outline and present this technique in such a way that the western reader can begin to practise it without significant prior knowledge.

This book is intended to guide readers through simple Shiatsu techniques, demonstrating how to employ them in order to carry out beneficial massage on the whole body. The book and video complement each other perfectly in that the sequence of movements is not only thoroughly explained but also demonstrated on video.

The text that follows is an introduction to the fascinating world of Shiatsu seen from my personal standpoint as a physiotherapist and medical practitioner. I hope that it will succeed in awakening your own interest and enthusiasm for Shiatsu.

Dr. Bernard C. Kolster

How to use the book and video together
The contents of both the book and the video are precisely coordinated and you will derive the greatest benefit from using them together. To gain a thorough understanding of and ability to use Shiatsu, you need certain basic elements of knowledge. You can read about these, in a much simplified and shortened form, in the first section of this book: "The theory of Shiatsu". You can then relax and watch the video. In this way you will acquire a good visual understanding of the applications explained in the second section of the book: "Practice". If after reading this section you feel the need to watch one of the more difficult hand movements again on the video, the camera icon in the margin are there to help you. Next to each of these there is a minute-count. This refers to the number of minutes into the video where each section of text is covered so that, using the timer on your video recorder, you will be able to find the corresponding sequence with ease. Simply run the video back to the beginning before use and set your minute-counter to zero, then fast-forward to the place indicated by the minute-count next to the camera icon.

Camera icon

The theory of Shiatsu: healing massage and the Far Eastern philosophy of life

What is Shiatsu?

Shiatsu is a method of healing through massage which originated in the Far East. In Japanese "Shi" means finger and "atsu" pressure; freely translated, "Shiatsu" therefore means "pressure with the fingers."

The roots of Shiatsu can be traced back to China to the time of the legendary "Yellow Emperor" (around 2000 BC). In the "Huangdi Neijing" – a collection of all the findings

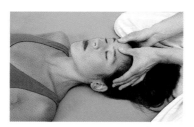

The word "Shi-atsu" comes from Japanese and means "finger pressure"

of the Chinese art of healing – certain massage techniques are described in conjunction with breathing exercises and herbal medicines. It is probable that Buddhist monks brought this knowledge to Japan more than a thousand years ago. Many hand movements and techniques were further developed in Japan and adapted to suit different cultural conditions, but it was only in the middle of the 20th century that Shiatsu was officially recognized in Japan as a healing massage.

In the meantime various styles of Shiatsu were developing with varying emphases. At the end of the 1970s the news of this healing massage spread to the west, especially to Australia and Europe, closely followed by America.

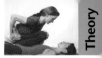

Philosophical and medical background

The basic principle of Shiatsu is: "Treat the whole person." This simple idea embodies the very philosophy of this ancient Far-Eastern healing art. The cosmos and all things and creatures within it are seen as one great unity. Every creature is in its turn a smaller "cosmos," that is to say a unity in itself which works as a whole and must therefore be seen as a whole.

For a better understanding of this philosophy, think of the human body as being like the mechanism of a clock within which there are many large and small cogs and levers. All the parts work together to drive the second, minute and hour hands. The energy to drive the clock comes from a spring that is wound up. If a single lever or cog gets out of balance, breaks, or comes loose, the whole system ceases to function and the clock stops. The clock-repairer then has to find out which of the small parts is responsible in order to fix the damage. Only when all the parts are working evenly once more will the mechanism start up again.

The body is like a complicated piece of clockwork machinery

Transpose this example on to the human body: as in the mechanism of a clock, all the organs and parts of the body work together. When one organ fails – e.g. the heart – the person affected dies unless help arrives in time. As mentioned above, a clock is driven by energy from a spring that has been wound up. When this energy has been used up, the spring loses its tension; the spring-like "vital energy" that drives the human body and sustains life is known in Japanese as "Ki," in China as "Chi" and in India as "Prana."

Ki – vital energy

Eastern philosophy maintains that each person receives a certain amount of vital energy at birth. This – to use the clock analogy once more – is the equivalent of the wound-up spring that provides the tension (energy) needed to drive the clock. When this tension has been used up, the clock won't work any more. In a similar way, when an individual's vital energy has all been used, that person dies.

"Ki" keeps us alive

The source of a person's vital energy is in the lower abdomen, known as the "Hara." The Hara plays an important role in Shiatsu (see page 17). From the Hara, vital energy – known as "Ki" – flows in an invisible stream through the whole body. When a person's whole body is permeated equally with vital energy, they are in the best of health. However, this is not usually the case as Ki is often unevenly distributed. Certain parts of the body have too much and others too little, and the resulting imbalance can lead to illness. Most people are only "semi-healthy" because their vital energy is unequally distributed. Shiatsu, properly applied, leads to a more equal distribution of energy, and so to increased well-being.

Vital energy flows through the body

The meridians

Like the water in a river, vital energy flows along invisible paths or "channels" through our bodies. In traditional eastern medicine, these channels are known as "meridians." These meridians are a fundamental part of the eastern art of healing. They cannot be seen or felt, but were described by Chinese healers more than 4,000 years ago. Modern scientists are finding more and more indications to confirm that these energy paths really do exist: for instance, they have found that the resistance of the skin is different at certain points on the meridians.

Twelve meridians are symmetrically arranged on either side of the body. Two further meridians (known as

The meridians in the body: front, back, and side

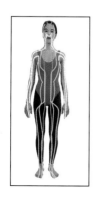 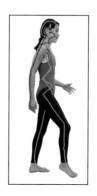 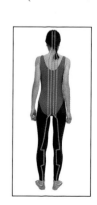

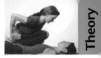

"exceptional vessels") run vertically down the very middle of the body, one at the front and the other at the back. Each meridian relates to a particular organ or area of the body. In the course of the day, vital energy, Ki, flows through one meridian after another.

Every meridian is related to an organ

The individual meridians

Each meridian has a specific role to play in the body. In the following list, the usual abbreviations for the various meridians are given in brackets.

- The lung meridian (LG) is responsible for the absorption of vital energy (which is universally present in the air) and for changing it into human vital energy. It governs the distribution of this energy throughout the body.
- The large intestine meridian (LI) regulates the absorption of water from food, and the excretion of waste from the body. It works closely with the lung meridian.
- The spleen and pancreas meridian (SP) plays an important role in digestion. It is responsible for the transformation of energy from food into the body's own vital energy, Ki.
- The stomach meridian (ST) initiates the digestion of food, drawing energy from it which then passes on to the spleen and the small intestine.
- The heart meridian (HT) regulates the circulation of the blood.
- The small intestine meridian (SI) is responsible for passing on the nutrients coming from the stomach. Nutrients and fluid are extracted from food in the small intestine. Fluid is drained off into the kidneys, leaving a thick pulp to pass into the large intestine.
- The kidney meridian (KD) stores Ki and distributes it to every organ. It also regulates the excretion of toxins.
- The bladder meridian (BL) regulates the storage and excretion of waste.
- The pericardium and circulation meridian, also known as the Heart Governor (HG), supports the functions of the heart and circulation.

- The Triple Heater meridian (TH) links the three centers of energy and distributes Ki throughout the body.
- The liver meridian (LV) regulates the storage of energy and nutrients in the liver and is responsible for breaking down toxins.
- The gall bladder meridian (GB) regulates the storage and transmission of the bile created in the liver, and works closely with the liver meridian
- The meridian known as the Governing Vessel and that known as the Conception Vessel may influence the other meridians. The former controls those at the back of the body and the latter those at the front.

Jitsu and Kyo

The human body is in an ideal state when vital energy, Ki, flows equally and unhindered through all of the meridians named above and there is, therefore, a harmonious balance of forces. The principle of Shiatsu is to find imbalances in the distribution of energy and use appropriate techniques to even them out. An excess of energy is called Jitsu, a lack of energy, Kyo.

Imbalance in the distribution of energy

Jitsu and Kyo are judged in terms of the state of the body as revealed by the flow of the meridians. The symptoms of Jitsu are stiffness, fullness and activity, whereas those of Kyo are weakness, emptiness and inactivity. Jitsu and Kyo can be diagnosed particularly well at certain points on the flow of the meridians: the Tsubos (see page 11).

For Jitsu states, a reduction in energy is needed in order to equalize its flow; for Kyo states, an increase in energy is required. The diagnosis of energy states, and the corresponding application of precisely targeted methods of healing, belongs to the higher level of Shiatsu. To reach this

Jitsu = excess of energy (demonstrated by: stiffness, fullness, activity)

Kyo = lack of energy (demonstrated by: weakness, emptiness, inactivity)

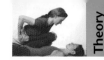

level requires instruction from an experienced Shiatsu teacher, but learning will be significantly easier if you have a firm grasp of the techniques and basic knowledge described in this book.

Tsubos

Tsubos are the points where Ki comes to the surface of the body. Various eastern methods of healing, like acupressure, acupuncture and Shiatsu, use these Tsubos to exert a healing influence on the flow of energy in the body. (They are also known and used as acupuncture points.) Most Tsubos are located on the meridians and take their names from these. To avoid any ambiguity, they are also designated by numbers. For example, "Bladder 10" denotes point number 10 on the bladder meridian.

If a person's Tsubos are over-sensitive, or even painful when touched, this means that there is a disturbance in the flow of energy. To relieve this, the sensitive points can be massaged using various techniques: pressing the Tsubos with the tips of the thumbs or fingers, for example. If you touch a sensitive Tsubo with the tip of your thumb you will get immediate feedback from the person you are massaging! They will experience the pressure as painful but not necessarily unpleasant. The recipient will often describe the sensation as spreading or flowing outward and, if they were to describe the direction it was flowing in, it would often correspond to the flow of the meridian to which the Tsubo belongs.

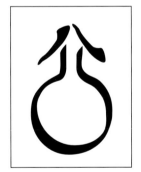

The Tsubo is depicted as a vessel with a lid

Yin and Yang

The two
opposing
forces of the
universeThe philosophy of the Far East recognizes two opposing forces that are the foundation of life and make it possible: these are known as Yin and Yang. In simplified terms, Yang is the creative and Yin the preserving force. To picture this, think again of a clock. The second hand jerks forward every second, driven by the tension in the spring – this is like Ki. The jerky movement corresponds to the Yang phase, the short pause before the next jerk, the Yin phase. Both phases are necessary to keep the hand moving round.

Now consider the heart: each heartbeat, via the blood, provides the body with the energy necessary to life. Like the mechanical ticking of a clock, the beating of the heart has two phases: first, the heart swells and fills with blood (the Yin phase); then it quickly draws inward, pumping the blood into the body (the Yang phase). Then the heart muscle relaxes again and takes in more blood (Yin phase) and so on.

Yin and Yang are symbolized by two intertwined shapes that, together, form a circle where one proceeds from the other. If one reduces, the other grows. But within this symbol another basic principle is illustrated. On the black plane there is a little white circle and on the white plane a black one. This means that one also contains the other: Yang is a part of Yin and vice versa.

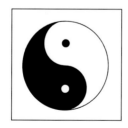

The symbol
for Yin and
Yang

However, Yin and Yang also represent pairs of opposites that complement each other. Yin embodies the creative, feminine, side with its feet on the ground, whereas Yang represents forward movement, action and dynamism. The pair of opposites, Yin and Yang, are also to be seen as separate aspects of the same whole. The principle of Yin and Yang permeates nature, as the table overleaf shows.

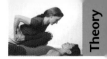

These are just a few examples, but they take us a step nearer to understanding the meaning of Yin and Yang. Naturally, this principle can also be applied to the body. The Yin and Yang cycles of the heartbeat have their equivalents

Yin	Yang
Woman	Man
Night	Day
Sleep	Wakefulness
Matter	Spirit
Stasis	Dynamism
Passivity	Activity

in breathing and all other physical processes. Inhaling is active, strong and dynamic, and therefore Yang; exhaling is passive and slow, and therefore Yin. The front of the body is Yang, the back, Yin. The meridians on the back are Yang, and those on the front Yin. So the meridians, the energy paths, are also governed by the principles of Yin and Yang. Accordingly this polarity principle influences the eastern art of healing. Indeed, the relationship of Yin and Yang is the entry-point for the understanding of many bodily processes, and consequently the key to a holistic approach to treatment.

Pairs of meridians

The meridians of the organs that are described as "hollow" (the stomach, small intestine, gall bladder, large intestine and bladder) belong to the sphere of Yang. The meridians of the organs that are used for "storage" (the kidneys, liver, spleen, pancreas, lungs and heart) belong to that of Yin. Each Yang meridian forms a unit with a Yin meridian, as follows:

- spleen and pancreas meridian and stomach meridian
- heart meridian and small intestine meridian
- liver meridian and gall bladder meridian
- kidney meridian and bladder meridian.
- lungs meridian and large intestine meridian

These combinations give us five important pairings which find their expression in what is known as the *five elements* system.

The philosophy of the five elements

The cycle and phases of transformation

The philosophy of the five elements describes the cycle of all things in the cosmos. Chinese philosophy starts from the premise that everything that happens – however small or large – has its place in the cycle of the five elements. The individual elements or stages are described as *phases of transformation.* Each phase of transformation has a particular element assigned to it.

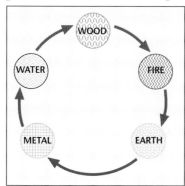

The cycle of
the five
elements

In this cycle, each element proceeds from another. So if, for instance, you were to apply the model to the seasons, the element *wood* would correspond to spring. *Fire*, which relates to great heat, would stand for summer and the element *earth*, in turn, would proceed from the glow of the fire, corresponding to late summer. Fall, the season of harvests, corresponds to the element *metal*. Winter, the season of rest, in which we consume our stores, is linked to the element *water*. Water is also the precondition for the birth of new life. In this way one element is "born" from another.

The cycle of transformation also applies to people and their relationship with the environment. For example, imagine you are planning to open a shop selling fashionable clothes. When you start out you have to deal with the planning and organization involved: you have to persuade a bank to put up the necessary money, you have to rent premises and think about the type and the quantity of things you want to sell. All of these ideas and plans are essential to the achievement of your goal although, so far, nothing concrete is in place. This phase can be assigned to the element *fire*. The next step comes when you have acquired the necessary finance, suitable premises and your merchandise. You then have the material with which you can work and do business; this material is symbolized by the element *earth*. Now you open your shop: people flock in, admire and buy your goods and the money jingles in the till. This state corresponds to the element *metal*. Then the routine of running a shop begins in earnest: the daily opening and closing, and the acquisition of merchandise. For this phase you will require endurance, strength and flexibility; this stage can be assigned to the element *water*. If you work very hard, your enterprise will eventually make a profit and this could serve as the basis for expansion; this phase corresponds to the element *wood* and closes the circle. Now, should you have any new ideas, you are ready to begin the next cycle.

As the above example makes clear, this model for the phases of transformation can be applied to all areas of life, all things and all living creatures.

The five elements are in evidence all around

One cycle follows another

The control sequence

As well as the cycle of transformation, in which one element proceeds from another, the five element system also has another set of interrelationships, known as the *control*

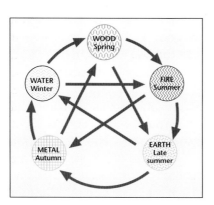

The elements control, and proceed from, each other

Pairs of meridians and the five element system

Pairs of meridians	Element
Liver/Gall bladder	Wood
Heart/Small intestine	Fire
Spleen and pancreas/Stomach	Earth
Lungs/Large intestine	Metal
Kidneys/Bladder	Water

sequence. The control sequence is based on the idea that the elements in the cycle also control and influence each other. So water controls fire, and likewise fire controls metal, metal wood, wood earth and earth water. Since each element is assigned to one of the pairs of meridians described above (see page 14) these too are included in the cycle of control.

The purpose of Shiatsu is to bring both those people receiving treatment and self-healers into line with this comprehensive system of universal order, outlined only briefly here. Shiatsu should be viewed as a mixture of healing system and philosophy.

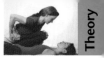

The Hara

Center of the body and source of vital energy

The term "Hara" may be freely translated as "lower abdomen," but it also has a deeper meaning than simply a description of a place in the body: in eastern philosophy it means the center of life. All the eastern martial arts, and other arts such as dancing, painting and music, as well as Shiatsu "come from the abdomen," from the Hara. This is the seat of physical equilibrium, of emotional and spiritual energy – vital energy. From the purely physical standpoint of weight, the area between the navel and the pubic bone is the body's center of gravity. The more low-lying it is, the greater the stability and equilibrium of the body. Conversely, the higher it is, the more unstable and insecure is the body's equilibrium.

The Hara is the center of life

Vital energy, Ki, is concentrated at a small point, around three fingers wide, below the navel. This point is known as the "Tanden." Vital energy emanates from this point and returns to it.

Movement from the abdomen

Before you begin a Shiatsu session, you should focus completely on your Hara. This will help you to enhance your internal equilibrium so that you feel rooted in yourself. When Shiatsu is performed correctly, all movements proceed from the Hara, and in order for this to happen effectively the Hara must be "open." The following exercise will help to make you conscious of your Hara and able to open it.

To be in inner harmony

Awareness exercise:
Learning to feel your Hara

Sit in an upright position – either on a chair or on the floor – sitting on your heels (see page 26).

Put one hand on top of the other, with the open palms turned upward in your lap. In this way your arms form a circle in which the energy can flow unhindered round your Hara.

Now focus all your attention on your breathing. With every breath try to breathe deeper into your abdomen, until you are breathing only with your abdomen. To make this easier, you can also place your hands on your lower abdomen. Now breathe "into" your hands. You will feel the rise and fall of your abdomen.

Breathing with the abdomen

Next, envisage yourself as breathing in and out of your Tanden (that is, your middle point, your center of gravity, the seat of your vital energy). Focus your consciousness and your whole spiritual energy on this point. Feel how every breath concentrates more energy there. You should feel the whole Hara, from the Tanden outward, become heavy and warm.

Warmth and light emanate from the Hara

Envisage the Hara opening and energy flowing out from it and into your body. Like a flower slowly unfolding, your Hara opens and warm light streams out of it and spreads through your whole body. Feel the warmth growing within you and become aware of the Hara as the source of this energy.

If your thoughts wander, do not feel pressurized to continue the exercise. Try to stay calm and focus your thoughts back on the exercise. If you can't manage to do this, simply try again another time.

Try to do this exercise as often as possible – preferably every day. Your awareness of your Hara will grow and your work with it will get easier.

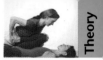

The hands

More than just a means of applying pressure

Like working from the Hara, working with the hands has a special meaning in Shiatsu. Your hands should be warm and smooth. Fingernails should be no longer than the tips of the fingers so that you do not hurt the person you are massaging. When performing Shiatsu remove all jewelry, particularly rings, bracelets and watches.

Strengthening, loosening, and warming

Using just a few simple exercises you can strengthen, stretch and loosen the muscles of your hands to prepare them for the treatment. To strengthen them, take a little rubber ball which you can easily get your whole hand around. Squeeze the ball and hold this tension for seven to ten seconds before letting go. Repeat this exercise ten times, then repeat with the other hand.

Strengthening the hand muscles

To stretch the muscles on the inner surface of your hands, place both palms together at chest height. Your elbows should point outward. Keeping your hands together, move them down a little way. You will feel a slight tugging on the muscles of your forearms. Hold this tension for 20 to 30 seconds and repeat the exercise three times. Next, stretch the flexor muscles of your hands and forearms. Place your palms on a wall at shoulder height and at shoulder width with straight, spread fingers and straight elbows. Now press your wrists on to the wall. While doing this exercise be careful not to raise your shoulders – keep them loose and relaxed.

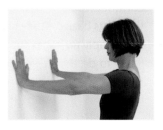

Stretching the muscles of the hand and forearm

You can increase the intensity of this stretch by raising your fingers and palm slightly away from the wall while keeping your wrists on the wall. You should experience a distinct, but not painful, pulling and stretching sensation. Keep this tension for 20 to 30 seconds before letting go. Repeat this exercise three times.

The energy of the hands

To increase the sensitivity of your hands, you might wish to complement your loosening and warming muscle exercises with the following simple but effective awareness exercise.

The first time your carry out this exercise, you may find it difficult to imagine the flow of warmth throughout your body. Remember, your hands must be warm; the more frequently you carry out this awareness exercise, the more refined your sensitivity will become.

Awareness exercise:
Feeling the energy in your hands
Shut your eyes and breathe in and out, calmly and evenly. Let your shoulders hang loose at your sides during this exercise.

Now hold out your hands in front of you so that the palms face, but do not touch, each other. Focus your attention on your palms. Try to feel the warmth that emanates from the palm of each hand in turn.

Feeling the energy in your hands

Now envisage this warmth as a stream of energy between your hands. When you can feel the stream of energy, begin to play with it: make very small, slow, circling movements in opposite directions. Increase the distance between your hands, but not so far that you can no longer experience the stream of energy and warmth.

Now it should be easy to imagine transferring this feeling of energy to your partner in the course of the Shiatsu massage described below.

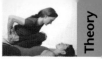

When not to use Shiatsu

Some general restrictions apply to the use of Shiatsu. It should not be practised when either the giver or the receiver:
- has just eaten a large meal
- has a fever
- has very high blood pressure
- is in the first three months of pregnancy.

Local problems such as wounds (including those arising from surgery) and inflammations that have not yet healed, varicose veins and areas affected by rheumatism should be avoided during treatment.

Only experienced therapists should treat people with serious health problems, such as a weak heart or cancer, and those people who have osteoporosis or epilepsy. During pregnancy certain meridian points should be treated with caution or not touched at all (please take note of all the advice given in the text). During pregnancy treatment is best carried out by an experienced therapist.

Be careful during pregnancy

Practice: giving and receiving Shiatsu

The fundamentals of Shiatsu presented in this book and video do not belong to any particular school. The choice of techniques and hand movements was guided by an aim to provide reliable access to this art and the satisfaction of achieving a successful outcome.

Using the book and the video together
If you have studied the principles of Shiatsu in the "Theory" section, and looked at the video, you will already have a good idea of the hand movements and massage techniques that are to be presented in this "Practice" section. As you read on, it will be easy for you to check any movement you are finding difficult on the video .

The camera symbols in the margin next to the description of particular techniques will enable you to find the corresponding sequence on the video, using the minute-counter on your video recorder. Simply run the cassette back to the beginning before use and set the counter to zero, then fast-forward to the place indicated next to the camera symbol.

In the practical section you will, first, learn the basic techniques of Shiatsu. These are simple massage movements that can be learned easily and used in many contexts. Once you have familiarized yourself with these basic techniques, you can follow the instructions in subsequent chapters and try out the first set of massages. It is essential to take note of the highlighted advice and precautions given with each application. After each massage there is a summary of how it can be used for various specific purposes.

Trying out the basic techniques and the first massages

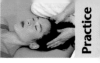

Note

Before you start the practical application of Shiatsu – and if this is your first experience with the subject – it is essential that you read the "Theory" section above. This provides important information which is vital to your understanding of the method and ability to carry it out correctly.

First master the foundations

How to perform Shiatsu

Room and atmosphere

 1:15

Shiatsu should be performed in an environment that is comfortable for both you and your partner (the person giving or receiving the massage). You need a calm room, in which you are sure you won't be disturbed. A pleasant atmosphere will really help you to relax. Muted or indirect lighting contributes to this, as does peaceful music (you must consult your partner's wishes about this). You should also make sure that you won't be interrupted by the telephone or the doorbell. You need enough space for the person receiving the massage to move around freely. You and your partner should wear comfortable clothes and remove all jewelry and other accessories. Clothing forms a warming envelope round the body that prevents too much energy being used just to keep the skin warm.

Create a pleasant atmosphere

What to lie on

 1:50

Shiatsu massage is carried out on the floor. The recipient lies on some form of mattress that is of a comfortable thickness without being too soft. A futon is an ideal choice, but several blankets placed on top of each other will do equally as well. It is preferable if the mattress is large enough for the person giving the massage to kneel on it next to the recipient.

The mattress should not be too soft

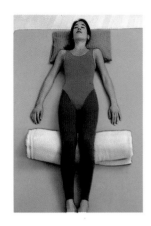

Put something comfortable under the head and knees

To encourage a relaxed lying posture use small, firm cushions or rolled or folded towels. If the recipient is lying on his or her back, place a rolled-up blanket under their knees. This will help to relax the abdominal muscles and back.

Before beginning Shiatsu, you must always remember to ask the recipient if he or she is comfortable.

2:15 ▶️ ## Massage from the Hara – preparing yourself

One of the most important principles of Shiatsu is to "work from the Hara." The Hara (the lower abdomen) is the seat

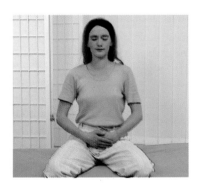

Focus on the Hara

of vital energy, Ki. Focus on your Hara when you carry out any of the movements. (This will be easier if you have carried out the Hara practice beforehand: see page 18.) It is also important that you breathe deeply and right down in your abdomen while carrying out the massage. This so-called "Hara breathing" helps you to retain a stable center of gravity as a basis from which to perform all further exercises and techniques.

Giving and receiving

Massage involves both giving and receiving. Try, as the giver of Shiatsu, to "feel yourself into" the recipient's body and to "see" with your hands rather than your eyes. This kind of massage will give you better feedback than almost any other procedure, enabling you to gauge the success of what you are doing. You will be able to tell from the degree of stimulation or relaxation of the recipient whether your Shiatsu massage is having the desired effect. If you use the correct hand movements, the recipient will quickly begin to relax and experience a sense of well-being, and you will be able to feel his or her tension melting away beneath your hands.

Be aware of the effect of the massage

Relaxation during Shiatsu massage

In order for your partner to be able to relax completely, you must also be relaxed and calm during the massage. So collect and compose your energies before you begin Shiatsu, and prepare to let them flow through your hands into your partner.

Concentrate on your Hara, and only begin to perform Shiatsu when you feel completely at peace within. Only then will you be in a position to devote your whole attention to your hands, making them sensitive to the body of the other person. The pressure of your hands will, after a while, attune itself to the condition of the receiver.

Pay attention to your hands

While carrying out a massage take care to remain relaxed. Do not hunch your shoulders, and always make sure you get into the best starting position for the next movement. If you are cramped you will miss out on the pleasure of practising Shiatsu. Working from the Hara prevents such tension from setting in.

Stay relaxed yourself

2:35 🎥 **Starting position**

The starting position for most techniques is for you to sit on your heels. You should kneel on the mattress with your bottom resting on your heels. In this position, the muscles in your thighs

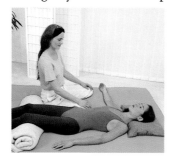

Starting position: sitting on your heels

will be slightly stretched. The further apart your knees, the more stable your position. While giving Shiatsu you should sit on your heels next to your partner. Move the arm they have nearest to you outward so that you have enough room to sit close to them. Before beginning the massage you should sit in this position for a while and focus on your Hara (see page 18).

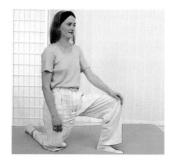

Kneeling up on one knee

From this starting position, you can then take up another important basic posture: kneeling on one knee, with one knee up and the other on the floor. There are numerous techniques that can be carried out from this position.

Working with your own body weight

Shiatsu depends on the optimal use of breathing and shifting body weight; it is not about sheer physical strength,

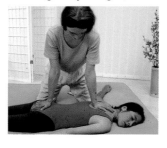

Making good use of your own body weight

so don't use brute force. Instead, work with your own body weight to apply precisely targeted pressure. In time, and with practice, you will learn how to carry out massage without exhausting yourself.

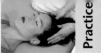

The right degree of pressure may be exerted by changing the position of your body. Pressure with the hands is applied by shifting the weight forward. Move from sitting on your heels to kneeling on all fours, bring your pelvis

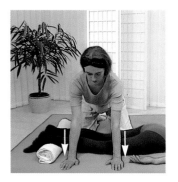

Shift your pelvis forward and put pressure on your hands

forward and shift the weight of your trunk to behind your outstretched hands. If you then move the weight of your pelvis back again, you will lessen the pressure on your hands. By leaning forward and back in this way you can judge accurately the amount of pressure you deliver. (Remember to work with straight arms.)

Applying pressure

Before carrying out a movement, get yourself into as near a right angle as possible to the area to be treated – this is the only way that you can make optimal use of your own body weight without exertion and avoiding the likelihood of twists and strains.

You should always exert pressure vertically on the area you are massaging because this encourages a precisely targeted working of the Tsubos. It also makes the most efficient use of your body weight and is kinder to your back.

Apply pressure vertically

You should always apply pressure slowly and in the same rhythm as your breathing. When the recipient exhales, "slip in" with your pressure. Then release the pressure until the next inhalation begins – between two and seven seconds (see page 31).

Working with both hands

In Shiatsu massage both hands are always in use. The resting hand (known as the mother hand or Yin hand) gives support and balance to the active hand (the child hand or Yang hand). Without continuous contact with the resting hand the recipient will feel uneasy during treatment. Visualize your hands as two poles: only when the two poles (i.e. both hands) are touching the body of the recipient can the vital energy, Ki, flow in a circle. When only one pole is in contact with the body, this circulation will be interrupted.

The hands are like two poles

Finding a harmonious rhythm

A Shiatsu massage is a continuous exchange between giver and receiver. So you should administer in it a harmonious rhythm. One treatment should flow on from the next so that the exchange is not interrupted. Be aware of your own breathing: it should be calm and even. Together, you and the recipient will gradually find your own rhythm.

One hand movement should lead straight on to the next

At first, these basic rules may seem complicated. But they all should come easily to you if you learn to work from the Hara. When you have carried out Shiatsu a few times, following the steps outlined, you will get more of a sense of what the above descriptions aim to convey. Listen to your inner self as you do the massage, work from your inside and observe the reactions of your partner. When both you and your partner feel at ease, you are doing it right.

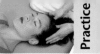

Summary: how to perform Shiatsu
- A pleasant warm room, free from distractions
- A thick, and not too soft, mattress or equivalent and small cushions to lie on
- Recipient lying in a relaxed, comfortable posture
- Massaging from the Hara – focusing on the Hara
- Relaxation during treatment
- Giving and receiving
- Taking up the right starting position: sitting on your heels or kneeling on one knee
- Exerting pressure by changing the position of your body
- Working with your own body weight
- Taking up a position at right angles to the part to be treated
- Exerting pressure vertically on the area being treated
- Pressing as the recipient exhales
- Always working with both hands
- Finding your own rhythm

Simple basic techniques

At present, countless variants of Shiatsu are being practised; each therapist evolves different techniques in the course of his or her work. With the basic techniques you will learn in the following sections, you will find it easy to carry out simple massage and to copy the examples of treatment that are covered.

Don't be discouraged if things don't work out first time. With practice you will be able to carry out all the techniques illustrated in the book and on the video.

Note:
In the following section, we describe Shiatsu techniques with reference to the people shown in the accompanying photographs. Although we refer to "she," Shiatsu is, of course, equally suitable for men.

2:45 ▶️📽

Pressure techniques

The application of pressure stimulates the vital energy, Ki, circulating in the energy channels (meridians). This means that pressure techniques are an important element of Shiatsu. There are many methods of applying pressure: using the thumbs, fingers, hands, elbows and other parts of the body. Certain general procedures need to be observed in order to carry out these techniques correctly (see page 29). The basic pressure techniques described below are those that you will use while carrying out the Shiatsu massage demonstrated later.

Degree of pressure and pressure points

Someone who is new to Shiatsu will probably wonder how pressure techniques are actually used: where, for how long, and how strongly pressure should be applied.

Pressure on the Tsubos

Generally speaking, pressure is applied at specific points, the Tsubos (see page 11). Most Tsubos lie on the energy paths, the meridians (see page 8). In order to start performing Shiatsu you do not need to know *exactly* where all these various points lie, so their precise location is only given in certain cases. In order to carry out the massages shown here, all you need to do is to follow the instructions and the corresponding pictures, using the video as a guide. The degree of pressure it is necessary to apply is determined by the sensitivity of the recipient, so ask them how they experience the pressure. You will also be able to feel how your partner reacts. If you apply too much pressure you will feel them tighten up or even stiffen convulsively.

When applying pressure, be aware of your partner's breathing

Be aware of their breathing: if you press so hard as to cause undue discomfort, they will involuntarily hold their breath, interrupting the calm, relaxed rhythm of their breathing. Below the threshold at which pain becomes unpleasant there is another sort of pain that is experienced as beneficial. This "beneficial pain" does not manifest itself in the signs described above, in fact it signals that the right degree of pressure is being delivered in the right place. It often radiates out along a meridian,

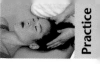

which is also a sign that the treatment is being delivered correctly. If you are using pressure techniques, do not start

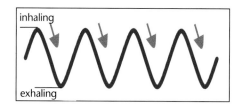

Pressure begins when your partner exhales

with the maximum pressure, but "slide" into it gradually: begin with gentle pressure as your partner begins to exhale, increase the pressure as they continue to exhale and then hold for two to seven seconds, or a complete cycle of inhalation/exhalation.

Advice on pressure techniques
- Always judge the amount of pressure you exert by monitoring your partner's well-being.
- Measure the amount of pressure you use with care. Older people in particular require only gentle pressure.
- Do not use pressure near to diseased or injured parts of the body.

🎥 3:05

Techniques using pressure with the heel of the hand
Pressure exerted with the heel of the hand produces a pleasant and deeply penetrating effect. A thoroughly relaxed hand is an important precondition for carrying out this technique effectively. Pressure is exerted with the heel of the hand by channelling your weight through your shoulders and outstretched arms.

wrong

right

wrong

right

Carry out a little practice exercise before starting on the first heel of the hand pressure technique. Your starting

Preparatory exercise: getting up from sitting on your heels ...

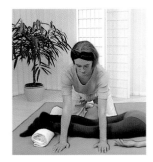

... and pressing on the mattress with the heels of your hands

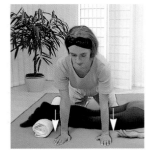

Heel of the hand pressure on the thigh

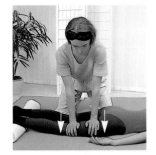

position should be sitting on your heels. Place both palms in front of you on the mattress.

From this position move forward on to all fours. You can consciously regulate the strength of the pressure that you exert with the heel of your hands on the mattress by pushing your pelvis and torso backward and forward. Keep your back straight and be aware of your Hara: breathe in through your lower abdomen and try to perform the movement from your Hara.

After this practice, carry out the heel of the hand technique on the back of your partner's thigh. Pressure should be exerted vertically on the mid-line of the leg.

Develop a feeling for how much weight you can apply. The pressure should not cause discomfort to the recipient (see page 30).

3:45

Thumb pressure technique

wrong

right

The thumb plays a very important role in performing Shiatsu. With it you can exert precisely targeted pressure on the Tsubos, the pressure points.

Apply the whole surface of the thumb, not just the tip (i.e. the thumb should be straight, not crooked). This technique may be quite a strain on your thumb at first attempt

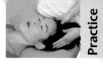

and will require some time to get used to it. Take your time and do not overtax yourself.

Exert an even pressure with your thumb on a single point. Avoid circling, sweeping or vibrating movements. As your partner exhales, build up the pressure steadily. As with the heel of the hand technique, you can regulate the thumb pressure by moving your pelvis and torso backward and forward.

Use the following preparatory exercise to develop a feeling for the thumb pressure technique. Sit on your heels. Place your two thumbs in front of you on the mattress, the other fingers extended for supporting the hand. Now move from this position on to all fours. By shifting your pelvis backward and forward you can shift your weight and so regulate the intensity of the pressure. For all pressure techniques, you must keep your arms, thumbs and fingers straight.

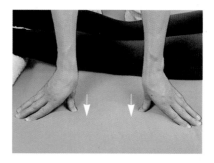

Thumb pressure on the mattress

After this preparatory exercise, start applying thumb pressure, as before, on the mid-line at the back of your partner's thigh. The pressure exerted should be an agreeable experience for your partner, and

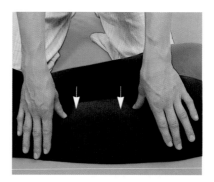

Thumb pressure on the thigh

should only be initiated, as with the other techniques, while the recipient is exhaling.

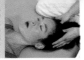
4:25

Finger pressure technique – "cleaning the wings"

"Cleaning the wings" is a very pleasant technique for treating tense shoulder muscles. For this technique your partner should be lying on her front, or – better still – on her side. With one hand, grasp the front of the shoulder and

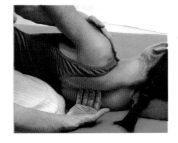

Move the hands toward each other

keep hold of it. Slide four fingertips of the other hand under the shoulder blade with the palm of the hand turned toward you. As your partner exhales, move both hands toward you, at the same time your fingers slide further under her shoulder blade.

This technique is excellent for relieving tension in the region of the shoulder blade. It should, of course, be an agreeable experience for the recipient.

4:50

Tiger's mouth grip

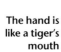

The hand is like a tiger's mouth

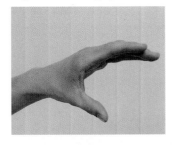

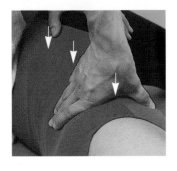

Pressing with the tiger's mouth on the side of the thorax

Using the technique known as the tiger's mouth grip you can stretch the sides of the body, exerting precisely targeted pressure at the same time. Hold your hand in a crescent, as though trying to grasp a bottle that is too large for you. From the side, the hand looks – with a bit of imagination – like the tiger's mouth from which its name is derived.

Your partner lies on her side. Lay your hand, fingers widely extended, on the side of her upper thorax. Shift your weight by

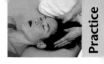

moving your pelvis back and forth, applying pressure with your hand at the same time. Apply pressure as your partner exhales, withdraw it as she inhales. Each time, place your hand a little lower down and repeat the cycle several times, pressing as she exhales, relaxing the pressure as she inhales. In this way work down step by step toward the pelvis.

Elbow pressure technique

 5:15

You can apply more intense pressure with your elbows than is possible with the hands. Consequently the elbow pressure technique is useful when larger groups of muscles are very tense. It also allows you to give your fingers and hands a rest. You can use your elbows on the shoulder, buttock, back and leg muscles. You should not, however, bend your elbows as far back as they will go, or they will be too sharp and the pressure will be painful for your partner.

To use your elbows on the shoulder muscles, stand or kneel behind your partner, who should be sitting or kneeling. Place your slightly bent elbows on her shoulder muscles between the neck and the shoulder joint; now press vertically downward, carefully. Begin when your partner is exhaling and gauge the amount of pressure to apply by asking how it feels to her. When you have finished, stroke her neck, shoulders and arms in a downward motion.

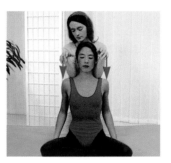

Press carefully with the elbows

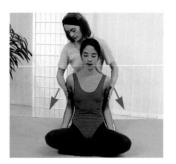

Afterwards, stroke the shoulders and arms

Be careful

Carry out the elbow pressure technique on older people only with the greatest sensitivity. It should not be used during pregnancy or on people with brittle bones (osteoporosis).

5:55

Stretching techniques

Stretching techniques are another important component of Shiatsu. They help to bring about relaxation, to relieve excessive build-ups of energy and thus assist in promoting the unhindered circulation of vital energy, Ki, throughout the body.

Release pent-up energy

There are multiple applications for stretching techniques in Shiatsu. The ones you will learn about below are not only simple but also important.

Stretching correctly

The basic principle of all stretching techniques is to extend the muscles to a point where the recipient feels a slight tugging sensation; never go beyond this point. Remember to keep your back straight and to breathe in and out from the lower abdomen.

Follow her breathing

When your partner exhales, you can gently intensify the stretch, but do not go so far that it becomes really painful. You can release slightly as she inhales. You should do this for five breath cycles, then replace the stretched limb in its normal position.

Do not make any sharp or sudden movements and avoid see-sawing as this will have the opposite of the desired effect. Instead of relaxing the stretched muscles, they become stimulated.

Notes on stretching techniques

- Carry out these stretches careful, especially with older people or where the limbs are very stiff.
- Do not perform any stretches on or near limbs that are injured or diseased.
- Be aware of your partner's individual pain threshold and do not exceed this point.

Stretching the back of the thigh

 6:15

Stretching the back of the thigh affects the bladder meridian. Kneel next to your partner's calves and get into a half-kneeling position with your outside foot next to her

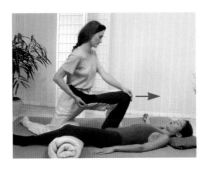

Push her bent leg toward the thorax

hips. Grasp her knee with your outside arm and her heel with your inside arm, and bend her leg.

Shift your weight on to the foot that is on the ground, and carry the leg you are holding with you into the bend. Hold the leg in this stretched position for three cycles of inhaling and exhaling.

As the recipient breathes out, intensify the stretch a little. If she pushes back, you have stretched too much. Finally, move to the other side, take up the half-kneeling position and perform the stretch on the other leg.

Stretching the arms

 6:40

The arms can be stretched in several positions, influencing the various meridians in this area.

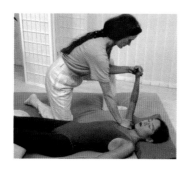

Loosen the shoulders by gently swinging the arm

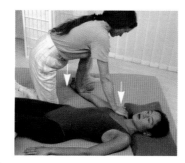

Stretching the arm, placed beside the body

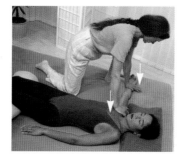

Stretching the arm, placed at right angles to the body

Before stretching, loosen the recipient's arm and shoulder muscles, operating from a half-kneeling position beside her. Place your right hand on her right shoulder, clasping the hand lightly with your left hand. Raise the arm off the mattress, with the elbow bent at a right angle. Next, swing the arm gently backward and forward. Your partner should try and let their arm be guided by you.

Now lay your partner's outstretched arm out to the side with the palm facing up and, with your right hand still resting on her shoulder, put the heel of your left hand on your partner's forearm, just above the wrist. Shift your weight forward on to your two hands, so that the muscles on the inner side of the upper arm and the forearm are stretched.

Finally, place your partner's outstretched arm at right angles to her body. Put your hands back in the same place as before, and shift your weight forward once more via your pelvis.

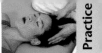

For the third position, sit on your heels sideways next to your partner's head. Take her arm, which is raised above her head, place it over your thigh and stretch it by pressing it with the heel of your hand, as in the first two positions. Do the same loosening and stretching procedure on the other arm.

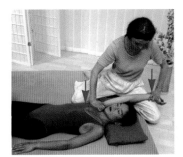

Stretching the arm above the head

Summary: basic techniques
Pressure techniques
- Pressure with the heel of the hand
- Pressure with the thumb
- Finger pressure – "cleaning the wings"
- Tiger's mouth grip
- Elbow pressure

Stretch techniques
- Stretching the rear of the upper thigh
- Stretching the arm

Massage

 7:55

The following section starts off by demonstrating a standard massage of almost the whole body. This activates vital energy and stimulates the powers of self-healing. You will already have learned the necessary hand movements in the section on basic techniques. Please remember that this is a massage and not a healing technique.

8:20

The bladder meridian

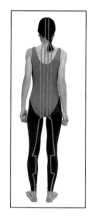

The bladder meridian goes all the way up the back

The bladder meridian is one of the 12 main energy paths and runs symmetrically up both halves of the body. Starting at the corner of the eye, it goes over the head and back down to the outside of the foot. At the nape of the neck it divides into two branches on each side. Many of the points you will work on in the massage that follows lie on the bladder meridian. These points play an important part in the treatment of backache and illnesses affecting almost all the organs of the body.

8:35

Back massage

As the supporting frame of the whole body, the back is particularly exposed to strain. There are many causes of back problems, whether they be the many everyday activities that make demands on the back, chronic bad posture or the wear and tear of age.

The back, an ideal place to practise

You can learn a great deal from a person's back. You can use almost every technique here and know at once whether your actions are succeeding. The back area is an ideal place to begin practising Shiatsu. Remember, however, to always get your partner to report their sensations as you massage. Many points you will work on in the back area lie on the bladder meridian.

The right way to lie

The recipient of a Shiatsu back massage should lie on their front. The head lies to one side and, from time to time, the recipient should turn it to the other side so that they do not get a stiff neck. You should be able to reach your partner comfortably from all sides.

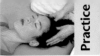

Notes on back massage

- The recipient should not lie on her front in the later stages of pregnancy.
- Do not lean on the spine while treating the back; only gentle pressure should be exerted here.

Concentrating on the Hara and making contact

 8:40

Sit back on your heels with your hips next to your partner's. First, focus on your Hara. Inhale and exhale consciously through your abdomen a few times, sinking into the center of your vital energy, Ki. Try to let everything to do with this massage come "out of your abdomen" (see page 17).

When you feel relaxed and ready, make contact with the recipient: place one hand between your partner's shoulder blades and the other hand on her sacrum. Leave your hands lying there for a moment, and feel the warmth coming from her body and its energy.

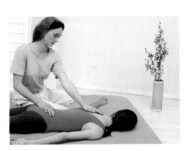

Your hands rest on her back

Heel of the hand pressure technique

8:55

Move from sitting on your heels to kneeling on one knee, and place your active hand on the recipient's upper back, next to the spine. The resting hand remains on the sacrum.

Apply pressure with the heels of both hands, shifting your weight forward over your pelvis and torso. Your arms are straight, and your hands have broad contact with

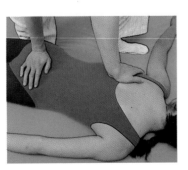

Pressure on the bladder meridian

the recipient's back. Press only when your partner is exhaling. Each time she inhales, move the heel of the upper hand a little way down. Apply only light pressure to the kidney region.

9:20

Thumb pressure technique with one hand

During the whole treatment the resting hand – the mother, or Yin, hand – remains on the sacrum. Now place the thumb

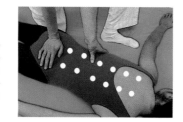

Move the thumb a little further each time she breathes in

of the active hand between the recipient's shoulder blades, about a thumb's width away from the spine. As she breathes out, shift your weight on to your out-stretched thumb. The pressure should be experienced as pleasant. In this Shiatsu technique, just as in heel of the hand technique, your active hand should move a step nearer to the recipient's sacrum each time she inhales.

10:05

Thumb pressure technique with both hands

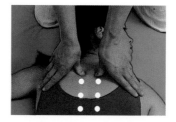

Pressure with both thumbs …

Sit on your heels at the end of the mattress nearest your partner's head. Place both of your thumbs just below the neck on both sides of the spine and along the bladder meridian. Again, press each time your partner exhales and move a little way toward the sacrum each time she inhales.

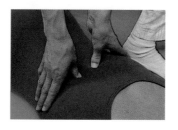

… on the bladder meridian

When you reach the highest point of the back, change positions and kneel up on one knee next to

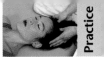
your partner's back. Place your thumbs between her shoulder blades and begin to move down again – in time with her breathing – to the sacrum.

Procedure: back massage
- Concentration on the Hara
- Making contact
- Heel of the hand technique
- Thumb technique with one hand
- Thumb technique with two hands

Techniques for the sacrum

 11:05

The sacrum is the base of the spine. It joins the left-hand and the right-hand pelvic bones, and forms the intersection between the mobile back and the almost immobile pelvis. The sacrum and the bones of the pelvis together form a very complex joint.

Painful lower-back problems often emanate from the area of the sacrum. The skin over the sacrum is also a reflex area for the bladder and the other organs of the lower body, so a massage in this area is very comforting when there is disease in these organs.

Lower back pain

Thumb pressure technique with both hands

 11:15

First, find the hollows in the sacrum with your thumbs: they are located two or three centimeters away from the center of the spine on either side. If you feel around with your thumbs to left and right, you will find four small dents down either side, one below the other. Your partner may get an "electric" feeling: this is because the nerves branching off from the spinal marrow are very close to the surface here.

Place your thumbs on the top two hollows and, with arms outstretched, shift your weight forward on to your

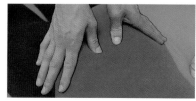

thumbs. Do not press down with the end of the thumb where the nail is, but with the flat surface (see page 32).

Feel for the perceptible hollows in the sacrum

As always remember to, apply pressure while the recipient exhales, moving forward, little by little, in the direction of the coccyx.

Heel of the hand pressure technique

11:30

Continue with your treatment of the spine by applying pressure with the heel of your hand. Now you are able to shift your weight forward more strongly.

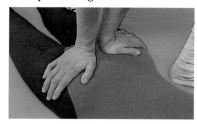

Apply pressure to the sacrum

Once again, press in rhythm with your partner's exhalations. Firm pressure on the sacrum is extremely relaxing and can often relieve pain.

Thumb circles

11:50

Thumb circles are a variant on the thumb pressure technique and enable you to extend your massage of particular points using a circular motion. Place your thumbs on both sides of

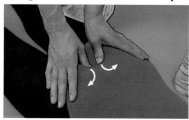

Push your thumbs outward in semi-circles

the center line of the coccyx, and push them outward in small semi-circles. Here too, you should gradually move downward with each semicircle.

"Pushing the sacrum together"

🎥 12:10

Now clasp you hands and lay them, still clasped, palms facing down on top of the sacrum. Everytime your partner exhales, press the heels of your hands toward each other over the sacrum. This massage offers relief and relaxation to a tense sacral region.

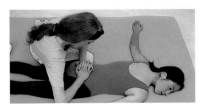

Push your hands together over the sacrum

Procedure: massaging the sacrum
- Thumb pressure technique with both hands
- Heel of the hand technique
- Thumb circles
- "Pushing the sacrum together"

Leg massage

🎥 12:25

The legs are the pillars of the body; they carry us through life and we may often feel the effects of wear and tear in our knee and hip joints. The muscles and sinews of our legs become hardened and can shorten as the result of an inactive lifestyle. This leads to an imbalance of energy, with too little in the legs.

There are six meridians running through each leg. Shiatsu stimulates the flow of energy along these. Regular Shiatsu massage also makes the muscles and sinews more flexible, promoting mobility and improving the circulation.

Stimulate the flow of energy

If you imagine your legs as pillars, then your feet form the solid base of these pillars, and indeed of your whole body. We stand and walk on our feet and our whole weight is loaded on to them. Forced from an early age into footwear that is usually too cramped, most feet lead what is, in view of their importance, rather a wretched and neglected life. Yet important meridians run through the feet; and, above all, the soles of the feet play host to reflex zones that are connected to all areas of the body. Give your feet the attention they deserve by including them in a relaxing Shiatsu massage.

For a leg and foot massage, the recipient should lie on her front. Place a rolled-up blanket under the ankles so that the knee joints are easily bent and the lumbar region is relaxed.

12:30

Heel of the hand massage technique

Place yourself on a level with your partner's knees, sitting on your heels. Then move into a half-kneeling position.

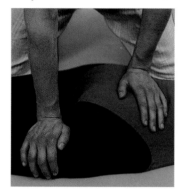

Move, step by step, toward the foot each time she inhales

Place your active hand on the center line of your partner's thigh, just below her bottom. The other hand (the mother hand) rests in a supporting position on the sacrum.

Move downward, step by step, along the bladder meridian toward the knee, applying pressure with the heel of your hand. Remember to exert pressure by shifting your body weight as your partner exhales. You can press the thighs quite hard, but avoid the back of the knees and use lighter pressure on the calves.

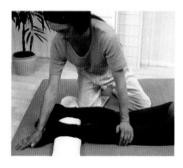

To conclude, stroke the soles of her feet

When you reach the heel, stroke the sole of the foot down to the tips of the toes a few times with the flat of your hand.

Thumb pressure technique with one hand

 13:15

Now work on the thigh, using the thumb pressure technique. With one hand again resting on the sacrum, place the other in the middle of your partner's thigh, on the bladder meridian. Shift your weight forward on to your thumbs as your partner exhales and move downward from one point to the next. Apply only the most gentle pressure to the back of the knee.

When you reach your partner's knees, move to the end of the mattress nearest to her feet and sit on your heels. Place your partner's lower leg across your own thigh, and loosen up the calf by rolling it vigorously to and fro. Continue to apply thumb pressure along the calf. Wrap your resting hand around the sole of your partner's foot and press gently each time you press with the other thumb. This will gently stretch the calf and also the bladder meridian. Finally, stroke the soles of the feet vigorously a few times with the flat of your hand.

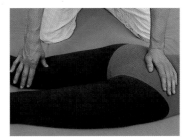

Pressing with your thumb, move toward her knee

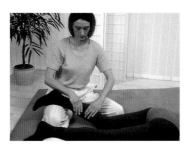

Work the calves

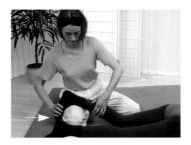

Continue thumb pressure on the calves

Be careful

The legs should not be massaged using pressure techniques if the recipient has varicose veins.

14:40 **Stretching**

Apply gentle pressure to the sole of the foot

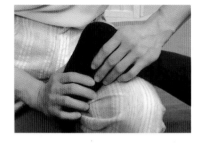

Stretch your partner's heel by exerting gentle pressure on the sole of her foot, while the other hand holds the leg at the heel.

Once again, the stretch is carried out as the recipient exhales and is held while she takes several breaths in and out.

Repeat, with the leg bent

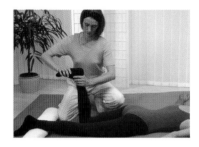

Now bend your partner's knee until the sole of her foot points to the floor. From this position stretch the heel again.

15:25 **Thumb pressure technique with both hands on the sole of the foot**

Apply pressure along the mid-line of the sole

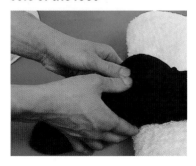

Place both thumbs on your partner's feet so that they are touching each other on the mid-line of the sole. Massage the sole using the thumb pressure technique moving from the heel to the beginning of the toes. Massage the other leg in a similar fashion.

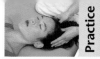
Pulling the legs

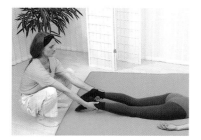

15:45

After massaging your partner's legs, grasp her feet around the ankle. Give both legs a gentle tug as your partner exhales by shifting your pelvis backward.

Shift your pelvis backward and pull gently

Stroking the feet

15:55

Finally, stroke both feet again with the flat of your hand.

Procedure: leg massage
- Heel of the hand technique
- Thumb pressure technique with one hand on the thigh
- Working the calves
- Thumb pressure technique with one hand on the thigh and simultaneous stretching of the calf
- Stretching the heels
- Thumb pressure technique with both hands on the sole of the foot
- Pulling the legs
- Stroking the feet

Shoulder and lateral neck muscles

16:05

The shoulders are the junction and the connecting link between the arms, the neck and the area around it, and the back. The three-way tension in this triangular zone frequently results in painful hardening of the muscles. Carrying out a simple Shiatsu massage in these areas releases tension and stimulates the flow of energy. The best position for massaging the shoulders and the area on each side of the

Release tensions

neck is with your partner seated or, as depicted here, lying on her side. Massage of the neck and the arms can then be performed with the recipient lying on her back.

How to lie
Your partner should lie on one side with her underneath leg outstretched and her upper leg bent up to the body for stability. (For increased stability you might like to lay a rolled-up towel in front of her abdomen and chest.) The bottom shoulder is turned slightly forward, with the arm bent close to the body. The head rests on a cushion so that the neck is stretched straight. You sit on your heels next to your partner's bottom.

16:10

Stretching the shoulder

Pull the
shoulders
gently
downward

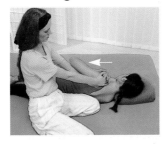

First, with the recipient lying on her side, stretch and loosen up the shoulder.

Place your partner's upper arm on your forearm. Enclose her shoulder in both hands and apply a gentle downward pull.

16:20

Circling the shoulder

Circle your
torso

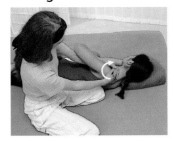

From the same position, move the shoulder joint in a circle. Make large circular movements so that the shoulder blade moves too. Follow through this movement with the whole top half of your body.

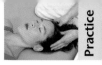

Stretching and stroking the lateral neck muscles

 16:40

Next, gently stretch the lateral neck muscles. Continue holding the shoulder with one hand, and stroke with the other, passing from the shoulder over the neck to the back of the head. Keep up a light stretch with the hand on the back of the head for a few seconds.

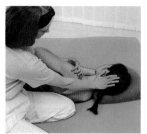

First stroke, then hold

"Cleaning the wings"

You can also loosen up the muscles under the shoulder blade with the "cleaning the wings" technique, with the recipient still lying on her side (see page 34). Hold the near side of her shoulder with one hand and, with the other, slide under her shoulder blade with the tips of your fingers. As she exhales, move both hands toward each other. Your fingers will glide under the shoulder blade and loosen the muscles in this area.

Glide your fingers under her shoulder blades

After "cleaning the wings," treat the other shoulder in the same way.

Procedure: massaging the shoulders and lateral neck muscles
- A stable lying position with straight neck
- Stretching the shoulders
- Circling the shoulders
- Stretching and stroking the lateral neck muscles
- "Cleaning the wings"

17:15

Abdominal massage

Little importance is attached to the abdomen in western society; according to the western point of view it "merely" houses the digestive organs. But in the philosophy of the Far East it has a much deeper meaning. There, the abdomen, or Hara, is seen as the site of vital energy, Ki. A healthy Hara is seen as a precondition for the health of the whole body (see page 17). The Hara massage demonstrated here will enable you to stimulate vital energy.

Massaging the Hara

How to lie

Massage of the abdomen, or Hara, is carried out with the recipient on her back. To relax the abdominal muscles, put a rolled-up towel under your partner's knees. Her head should rest on a flat cushion.

Note:

Most people have a very sensitive abdomen, so be particularly careful, especially in pregnancy or when the recipient has abdominal problems.

17:30

Making contact

First, make contact with your partner. Lay one hand directly on her abdomen, over the Hara, and leave it there for a few moments.

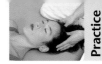

Circular stroking

Now place both hands flat on her abdomen and perform slow, circular, stroking movements in a clockwise direction over the Hara. The circles should gradually grow wider.

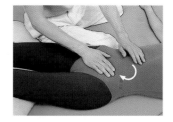

 17:40

Stroke in circles over the Hara

Cat's paws

Next, let your fingertips wander clockwise once or twice round her navel, as though they were cat's paws.

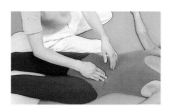

18:00

Move around the navel

Deeper breathing

Now lay one hand on the lower abdomen, the other on the upper abdomen. Slide the upper hand, little by little, from the upper abdomen up over the breastbone to the base of the neck. Each time the recipient inhales, move your hand a little further up; and, as she exhales, leave it motionless. This exercise has a calming effect and will also help your partner to breathe more deeply.

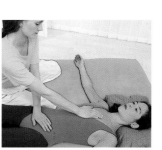

18:15

Place your hands without pressing

Practice

18:40

Stroke, then let your hands rest

Taking leave

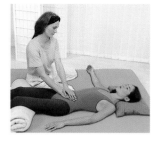

Before taking leave, stroke your partner slowly and gently from thorax to abdomen several times with alternating hands. Allow your hands to rest briefly on the abdomen before ceasing contact.

Procedure: massaging the abdomen
- Lying with the abdominal muscles relaxed
- Making contact
- Circular stroking
- Cat's paws
- Deeper breathing
- Taking leave

19:00

Arm massage

Whereas the legs enable us to stand firm and move forward, the arms help us to communicate. They gesticulate, welcome and embrace. The arms' radius of action is significantly greater than that of the legs. But, as with the legs, there are six meridians running through each of them. If you are to massage your partner's arms, she must "let go" – this means relaxing, loosening up, becoming passive. Many people find this very difficult, so in order to initiate arm massage and enable your partner to loosen up, it is necessary to perform movements with her arms that allow her to remain passive.

19:10

Loosening up
To loosen your partner's arms, shake them slowly and gently. Sit on your heels next to her. Lay one hand on her shoulder joint and use the other to lift her arm by the wrist,

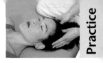

so that it is slightly bent at the elbow and moves freely and loosely at the shoulder. Move the arm backward and forward with a gentle rocking motion (see page 38). Your partner should consciously allow her arm to be guided through these movements while she remains passive.

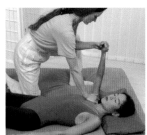

Circling

 19:20

Finally, rotate and extend the arm. This is done by holding it at the wrist and moving it away from you and above the recipient's head. Crook the arm and bring it back toward you so that the elbow describes a circle. One hand remains on the shoulder joint the whole time. Repeat this exercise several times.

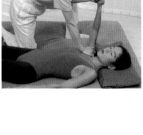

Loosen the arm by rotating it

Heel of the hand pressure technique

 19:35

Now place the arm with palm uppermost, at right angles to the recipient's side, and massage the inner side of the arm using the heel of the hand pressure technique. The active hand moves from her shoulder, pressing gently all the time, down the arm, while the passive hand rests on her wrist. The inside of the elbow is sensitive, so do not exert any pressure there.

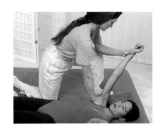

Move along the arm step by step

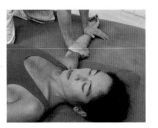

20:10

Apply pressure
with the
thumb, point
by point

Thumb pressure technique

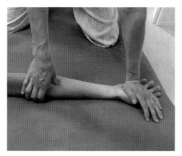

Now use thumb pressure in the same way as you used the heel of the hand pressure, following the mid-line point by point from the shoulder to the palm and, as before, avoiding the inside of the elbow.

Procedure: arm massage
- Loosening
- Circling
- Heel of the hand pressure technique
- Thumb pressure technique

20:55

Hand massage

Our hands are our most important tools. Their tasks might be described as giving, receiving and doing. Without their capacity for performing different movements, human civilisation – i.e. scientific and technical progress – would be inconceivable.

The hands, our
most important
tools

There are many reflex zones on the hands (as on the feet) that are connected to other parts of the body. Three meridians begin and end on the fingertips of each hand. So Shiatsu massage on the hand can, like that on the foot, be a very intense experience.

How to lie

Your partner lies on her back, as with arm massage. But if you are doing hand massage alone, she can sit. Take your partner's hand in both of yours.

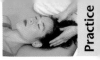

Stroking the palms and the fingers

20:55

Begin by applying a few soft strokes of the palms and the fingers. Take one of your partner's hands and hold it gently in yours. Initiate the massage by stroking the whole hand.

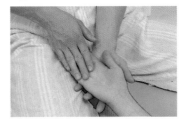

Gently stroke the palms of the hands

Finally, while continuing to hold her hand, use your thumb and index finger to stroke each individual finger from the joint to the finger tip.

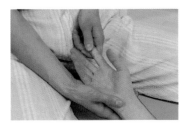

Stroke the fingers

21:45

Pulling the fingers

Hold the bottom joint of each finger with your thumb and index finger, and use your other hand to gently pull at each finger joint. Do this to every individual finger.

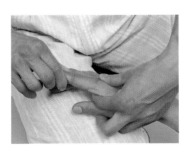

Pull each finger gently

21:45

Thumb pressure on the back of the hand

Apply light pressure, point by point, with your thumb to the space between the middle bones on the back of the hand. When performing this technique you can bend the thumb slightly so as to get between the bones.

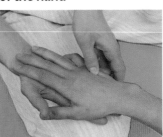

Press in between the bones of the hand

22:10

Stretching the palm of the hand

Threading your fingers together ...

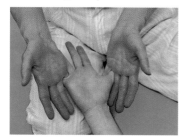

Now turn the hand palm-upward again, and hook one of your little fingers into the space between her thumb and index finger, and the other into the space between her little finger and her ring finger.

... and stroking outward with your thumbs

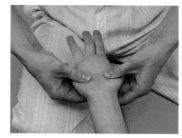

Your index, middle and ring fingers press the back of your partner's hand, and your thumbs stroke her palm, pressing gently, from the middle to the outside. In this way you gently stretch her palm.

Your thumbs should begin at the wrist and advance with every additional stroke a little nearer to the bottom joints of her fingers.

Stroking

22:45
Finally, stroke the inside and the outside of her hand a few times as you did at the beginning of the massage, using the palm of your hand.

> **Procedure: hand massage**
> - Stroking the palm and the fingers
> - Pulling the fingers
> - Thumb pressure technique on the back of the hand
> - Stretching the palm
> - Stroking the hand

Neck massage

 23:05

The nape of the neck is the connecting link between the head and the back. The neck vertebrae which join the head to the back allow the head a great deal of mobility. Faults in posture, as well as psychological burdens ("What a pain in the neck!") and many other causes can produce painful tension in the muscles that can limit this mobility to an immense degree. Pain in the nape of the neck can be set off by the slightest movement and is almost as bad as toothache. A very simple Shiatsu massage will loosen up the muscles, stimulate the flow of energy and produce a feeling of "lightness."

When the nape of the neck is tense and stiff, it hurts

How to lie
Your partner should, once again, lie on her back, but you should remove the cushion from underneath her head. Sit on your heels at the end of the mattress nearest to her head.

Taking the head in both hands

 23:10

Gently slide your hands underneath your partner's head near the nape of the neck, and carefully roll it to one side then the other. Now allow her head to lie still in your hands.

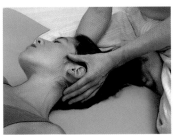

Stroking with two hands

23:15

Now apply strokes from the nape of the neck to the back of your partner's head with the palms of your hands.

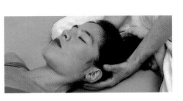

Giving and receiving Shiatsu 59

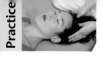

 23:40

Stroke the nape of the neck and the back of the head

Stroking with one hand

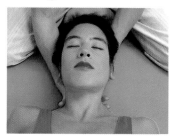

Take hold of the nape of your partner's neck in one hand, and carry out single-handed stroking movements, one hand after the other; you can pull slightly.

Procedure: neck massage
- Recipient on her back without a head cushion
- Taking the head in both hands
- Stroking with two hands
- Stroking with one hand

 23:55

Head and face massage

For many people, the most relaxing and enjoyable part of a Shiatsu massage is the treatment of the head and face. Many meridians have a relationship to the head and face, and Shiatsu harmonizes and regulates the flow of energy in these meridians. A pleasant side-effect is that massaging the face removes the tension from the facial muscles and makes the recipient look relaxed and beautiful.

Harmonizing the flow of energy

How to lie
Your partner lies the same way as for massage of the muscles round the nape of the neck: on her back, without a pillow and her head directly on the mattress. You sit on your heels at the end of the mattress nearest to her head. Take your time when massaging the head and face.

Thumb pressure technique – the bladder meridian

 24:05

Place the thumbs of both hands about two centi-meters away from the center line of the recipient's scalp, just at the hairline. Then, applying thumb pressure, move them along the bladder meridian to the back of the head.

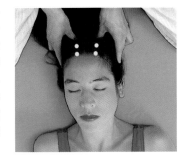

Press the bladder meridian, point by point …

Thumb pressure technique – scalp mid-line

 24:30

Next massage points along the center line of the head with one thumb on top of the other. Once again, move from the hairline to the back of the head.

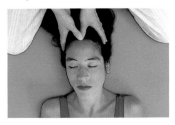

… and the mid-line of the scalp

Stroking the face

 24:45

First, massage the face with gentle stroking movements of the thumbs. Begin at the forehead: place your thumbs on the middle of your partner's forehead, then move them, with only the gentlest pressure, out across the temples.

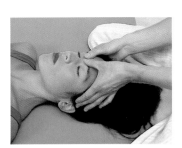

Stroke outward with your thumbs, over the forehead …

Treat every part of the face in this same way: first the eyebrows, then the under-eye region, then the cheekbones, the upper jaw and, finally, the chin area.

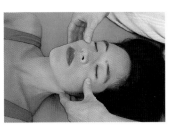

… and over the cheeks

23:25

Two-handed thumb pressure technique on the face

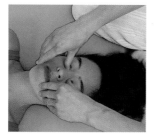

Press the points with your thumb ...

After stroking the face, carry out a pressure massage with your thumbs. Progress from one point to the next along the lines that you stroked from the center outward, over the eyebrows, in the area below the eyes, beneath the cheekbones, over the upper jaw and the chin.

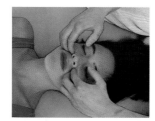

... or with your fingertips

The region below the cheekbones can be pressed with the fingertips held close together rather than the thumbs.

26:40

Placing the hands on the ears

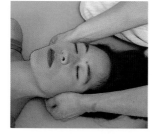

Deepen her relaxation

To conclude the head and face massage, place both palms over your partner's ears. This will deepen the relaxing effect of the face massage. Take your hands away very slowly.

Procedure: head and face massage
- Lying down, with no head cushion
- Thumb pressure technique – bladder meridian
- Thumb pressure technique – scalp mid-line
- Stroking the face
- Two-handed thumb pressure technique on the face
- Placing the hands on the ears

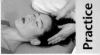

Ending the massage

27:00

Conclude the massage by placing your hands on your partner's abdomen. Leave them there for a few breaths.

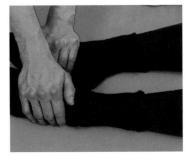

Finally, place your hands on the front of her feet and then take your leave.

Shiatsu leads to a feeling of deep and pleasant relaxation; give

Finally, lay your hands on the backs of her feet

your partner time to enjoy this wonderful feeling. After a whole-body massage, the recipient should take a rest of 10 to 15 minutes. An important point to remember is to cover her with a blanket to stop her getting cold.

The deeply relaxed feeling can noticeably outlast the rest period, so let the recipient know about this and warn her to be particularly careful in traffic and while going about her daily business.

Rest, and look out for physical reactions

Remember also that there can be physical reactions to Shiatsu; these include profound tiredness, restlessness, or symptoms such as fever, slight shivering, or even diarrhea. These reactions are positive signs and show that the body is responding to the Shiatsu it has received; they will disappear on their own.

Before your next session, ask your partner to tell you in detail about her experience of the treatment and to let you know whether anything out of the ordinary happened that might be connected with the massage.

Practice

Procedure: ending the massage
- Let your hands rest on the abdomen
- Place your hands on the front of the feet
- Allow time for rest (cover your partner with a light blanket to keep her warm)
- If your partner is feeling drowsy, suggest that she does not drive or operate machinery until she feels fully alert
- Refer to the possibility of spiritual and physical reaction

Summary: massage
- Back massage (page 40)
- Techniques involving the sacrum (page 43)
- Leg massage (page 45)
- Massaging the shoulders and neck muscles (page 49)
- Abdominal massage (page 52)
- Arm massage (page 54)
- Hand massage (page 56)
- Massaging the nape of the neck (page 59)
- Head and face massage (page 60)
- Ending the massage (page 63)

64   **Giving and receiving Shiatsu**

Applications

🎥 27:35

Hara massage for exhaustion

🎥 28:00

A Hara, or abdominal, massage is a pleasant and relaxing way to overcome exhaustion and it is easy to do. Once again, the recipient should lie on her back (see page 24).

Getting in touch with the rhythm of her breathing

First, place your hand on the recipient's abdomen and weigh it down with your other hand. Use both hands to get in touch with the rhythm of her breathing.

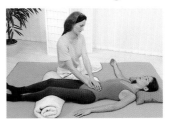

Rest your hands on the Hara

Moving around the navel

Move your two hands, one on top of the other, clockwise round the navel. Go a bit further round each time she inhales, keep them still while she exhales.

Circular stroking

Now lay both hands flat on her abdomen and perform gentle, clockwise circling movements.

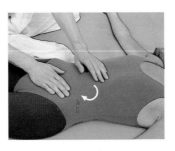

Stroke gently in circles over the Hara

Pressure with the heel of the hands

Move your hands in a clockwise direction

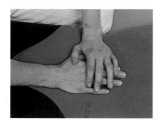

Both hands are now lying, one partially under the other, on the navel. Use the heel of the hands to exert very gentle pressure on the abdomen. Perform clockwise pressure movements around the navel.

Cat's paw

Move your fingertips like a cat's paws in a clockwise direction round the navel (see page 53).

Stroking

Use both hands one after the other to stroke the center line from chest to abdomen and downward toward the navel (see page 54).

Taking the abdomen between your hands

Feel her breathing

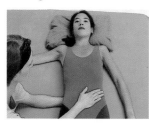

Next put one hand under your partner's back, while the other hand remains at the level of her navel for the duration of several breaths. Try to sense the abdomen between your hands.

Circling round the navel

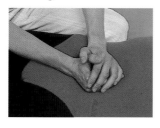

Clasp your hands loosely over your partner's abdomen, and make clockwise circling movements round the navel, touching the body only with the edges of your hands.

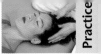

Ending the massage

To end the massage, rest quietly for a little while with both hands on top of the abdomen.

Procedure: Hara massage for exhaustion
- Getting in touch with the rhythm of her breathing
- Moving round the navel
- Circular stroking
- Heel of the hand pressure
- Cat's paw
- Stroking
- Taking the abdomen between your hands
- Circling round the navel
- Ending the massage

Self-massage for headaches

 30:00

Headaches can often be brought on by tension in the muscles of the nape of the neck.

Simple self-massage techniques can bring relief. Sit or stand upright, holding your back straight. Focus your concentration on the rhythm of your breathing: breathe calmly and evenly from the abdomen.

Stroking the neck

Stroke the nape of your neck and the area around it calmly but firmly a few times with both hands, beginning at the back of your head.

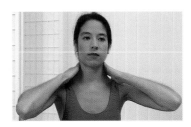

Stroke the nape of the neck and the shoulders

Kneading the shoulder muscles

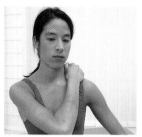

Then knead the muscles of one shoulder with the palm of the opposite hand. Move from the base of the neck across the shoulder to the muscles of the upper arm. Repeat several times, then massage the other shoulder in the same way.

Thumb pressure technique at the back of the head

Points: "Bladder 10" and "Gall bladder 20"

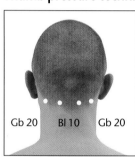

Gb 20   Bl 10   Gb 20

Search round the back of your head on both sides with your fingertips for the edge of the skull, which you should be able to feel quite easily. Now feel with your thumbs for the sensitive spots just under it. On both sides of the central line there are pressure points for the bladder meridian ("Bladder 10"), and a little further to the side, for the gall bladder meridian ("Gall bladder 20").

Exert pressure on each of the individual points by leaning your head back on your thumbs. Hold the pressure, with head bent back, for one breath cycle. Rest and repeat several times.

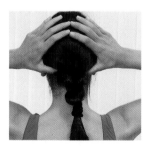

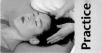

Pressure technique for the face

There are some effective pressure points on the face as well. At the level of the nostrils, directly below the pupils, you will find "Stomach 3" on the stomach meridian. Apply gentle pressure to this point with your middle fingers.

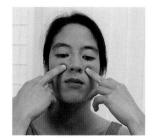

Press point "Stomach 3"

Put your palms together and apply pressure to the point between your eyebrows with your middle fingers. Try to relax inside and breathe calmly.

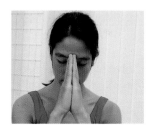

Pressure technique on the hand

Another point that is effective for headaches ("Large Intestine 4") is in the hand. You can find this point by placing the thumb and index finger together. This leads to the protrusion of a small lump of muscle, and the point you need is at the top. Press it as hard as you wish to without hurting.

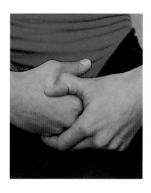

Press point "Large intestine 4"

Point massage on the back of the foot

You can also massage a point on the top of your foot, "Liver 3", which has, among others, a relaxing effect. Do this massage with your heel.

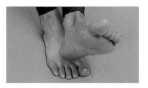

Massage point "Liver 3"

Circling on and stroking the temples

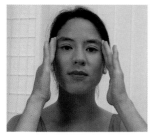

**Gently circle
and stroke**

Making circling and stroking movements on the temples with the fingers is both beneficial and relaxing. First, place your index, middle and ring fingers on both sides of your temples and apply gentle pressure with a circling motion. Then, with the fingers close together, stroke down from the temples. Press as hard as you wish to without hurting.

Procedure: self-massage for headaches
- Stroking the nape of the neck
- Kneading the shoulder muscles
- Thumb pressure on the back of the head
- Pressure techniques on the face
- Pressure techniques on the hand
- Massaging points on the back of the foot
- Circling on and stroking the temples

32:20 ## Massage for menstrual problems

Shiatsu can also help to relieve period pains, either in someone else or yourself (see page 75).

Rocking the pelvis

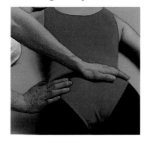

**Rock the pelvis
to and fro**

The recipient starts off by lying on her front. Gently rock her pelvis back and forth in this position. One of your hands should rest on her hip, the other on her sacrum; this hand can move up and down her back as you rock.

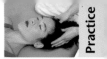
Stretching the back

Now stretch her back. One hand rests on her sacrum, the other between her shoulder blades on the spine. You carry out the stretch by gently shifting your weight on to the heels of your hands and pressing your arms outward.

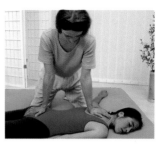

Apply pressure with the hands: on the mid-line …

Repeat this stretch several times, putting your hands on the pelvis and the shoulders, so that you also exert a sideways and a diagonal stretch. Be careful not to let your hands slip off.

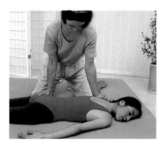

… sideways and diagonally

Heel of the hand pressure technique on the sacrum

Now exert pressure with the heels of your hands to the left and right of the mid-line in the sacral area (see page 44). Vigorous pressure here can bring substantial pain relief.

Thumb pressure techniques on the sacrum

Next, apply pressure with your thumbs to the hollows in the sacrum (see page 43).

"Pushing the sacrum together"

Now join your hands, lay them on the sacrum and push the heels of the hands together (see page 45).

Rubbing the sacrum

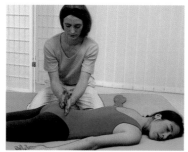

Vigorous rubbing produces a pleasant sensation of warmth

With the edges of your hands on the sacrum, rub your palms together briskly, applying some pressure to the sacrum. This creates a pleasant feeling of warmth in the pelvic region.

Pulling the legs

Squat by your partner's feet, take hold of her ankles and pull gently on both legs by shifting your weight backward (see page 49).

Walking on the soles of the feet

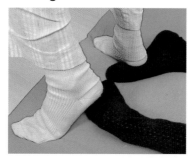

Carefully "walk" on her feet

Take away the rolled-up blanket from under your partner's ankles, and place the tips of her toes together. Now turn your back to her and stand with your heels on the soles of her feet, your toes facing outward. Move along the soles of her feet, but not on to the toes. This technique must not be at all painful or unpleasant for your partner, so be very gentle and careful. When you have finished, remain standing on the soles of her feet for a few moments.

For the massages that follow, your partner should turn on to her back (see pages 23–24 for how to prepare for Shiatsu).

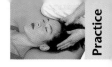

Circling the legs and loosening the sacrum

Take both of your partner's bent legs between your knees, hold them tightly on the outside of the knees and perform rotating movements with them. In this way the tense sacral region can be massaged gently and mobilized.

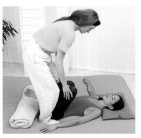

Perform circular motions with her legs

Stretching the thighs and massaging points on the legs

Starting from the above posture you can stretch the thighs and relax the pelvis from various positions. First, bend your partner's legs more tightly, and hold them in this position for a moment.

Next, stretch out one of her legs and bend the other, placing the foot on your thigh. Move the knee toward the head and, at the same time, apply thumb pressure to the "Spleen/Pancreas 6" and "Stomach 36" points.

You will find "Stomach 36" four finger-widths below the kneecap on the outer edge of the shin bone (see page 75), and "Spleen/Pancreas 6" four finger-widths above the inner ankle bone (see page 76).

Simultaneously, stretch "Spleen/ Pancreas 6" and press "Stomach 36"

Circling the ankle joint

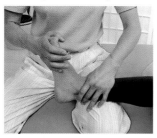

Stretch your partner's bent leg, then sit back on your heels and place her leg on top of your thigh. Clasp her lower leg with one hand, her foot with the other, and circle the ankle joint.

Point massage on the back of the foot

Press "Liver 2" and "Liver 3"

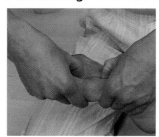

Look for the pressure points, "Liver 2" and "Liver 3," between the first and second bones in the middle of the foot (see page 76). Gently press both of the points simultaneously with your thumb.

Meanwhile, straighten the legs by gripping your partner's ankles and pulling gently (see page 49). After this, carry out the stretch, the ankle circling and the point massage on her other leg; finally, pull both legs straight.

Elbow pressure technique on the soles of the feet

Lean on her carefully

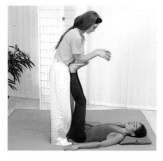

Bring your partner's legs into a vertical position, with knees extended, and lean them against your body.

Rest your elbows, bent at right angles, on the forward part of her soles and shift your weight on to them.

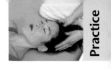

To conclude, put down her legs carefully, supporting them behind the knees. Take your leave by laying your hands on the tops of your partner's feet.

Procedure: massage for menstrual problems
- Rocking the pelvis
- Stretching the back
- Heel of the hand pressure technique on the sacrum
- Thumb pressure technique on the sacrum
- Rubbing the sacrum
- Pulling the legs
- Treading on the soles of the feet
- Circling the legs and loosening the sacrum
- Stretching the thighs and massaging the legs
- Circling the ankles
- Point massage on the back of the feet
- Elbow pressure technique on the soles of the feet
- Laying your hands on the back of the feet

Self-massage for menstrual problems

 38:15

You can treat period pains effectively yourself with the specific application of Shiatsu massage techniques to various pressure points.

Get into a comfortable sitting position, on the floor if possible. Use a cushion if you wish.

Massaging the "Stomach 36" point

Place the soles of your feet on the ground. Search for the "Stomach 36" point on the outside edge of the shin bone (see p. 73), press the point on both legs with your thumbs.

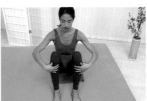

Press "Stomach 36"

Massaging the "Spleen/Pancreas 6" point

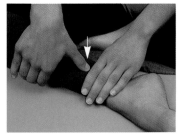

"Spleen/
pancreas 6"
lies a hand's
width above
the ankle

Place the soles of your feet together. Locate the "Spleen/Pancreas 6" point by placing the little finger of one hand in the center of the ankle bone on the opposite foot. You will find the point near the index finger of your hand, on the back edge of the shin bone (see page 73). Massage this point on both legs by pressing with the thumbs.

Massaging the "Liver 2" and "Liver 3" points

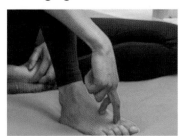

"Liver 2" and
"Liver 3" lie on
the back of the
foot

"Liver 2" and "Liver 3" are located on the back of the foot, between the first two middle bones. Press both points simultaneously with the index and middle fingers.

Procedure: self-massage for menstrual problems

- Massage point "Stomach 36"
- Massage point "Spleen/Pancreas 6"
- Massage points "Liver 2" and "Liver 3"

Learning about Shiatsu in more depth

You will by now have a good impression of the spiritual foundations of Shiatsu, and you have learned a few possible applications. One of the great advantages of Shiatsu is that its simple basic techniques can be learned quickly by the non-professional. It is to be hoped that, through the use of this book and video, you too will experience the benefits this type of massage can bring.

Shiatsu is, however, a comprehensive method of healing and treatment; the precise application of it to ailments and disturbances of the system requires a broader knowledge than it is possible to give here. If, after this introduction, you feel that Shiatsu suits you and that you would like to find out about it in more depth, you would be well advised to embark on a Shiatsu course. Please note that to be able to apply Shiatsu with precision as a method of healing requires personal and detailed training by an experienced teacher.

Learn Shiatsu as a method of healing

Appendix

Further reading

Cowmeadow, Oliver. Shiatsu – A Practical Guide. Element Books Limited, Shaftesbury, UK/Element Inc, Boston, USA 1998.
Liechti, Elaine. Shiatsu – Japanese Massage for Health and Fitness. Element Books Limited, Shaftesbury, UK/Element Inc, Boston, USA 1992 (reprinted 1997).
Liechti, Elaine. The Complete Illustrated Guide to Shiatsu. Element Books Limited, Shaftesbury, UK/Element Inc, Boston, USA 1998.

Other videos in this series
Kolster, Bernard C.: Partner Massage. Cologne, 1999.
Kolster, Bernard C.: Reflexology. Cologne, 1999.
Kolster, Bernard C.: Look after your Back. Cologne, 1999.
Kolster, Bernard C.; Cernaj, Ingeborg: Balance. Cologne, 1999.

About the author

Bernard C. Kolster is a doctor of medicine and a physiotherapist. He has been involved, for many years, with the study of whole-body treatment, rehabilitation procedures after serious illness and operations, eastern medicine, and natural healing. In recent years Dr. Kolster has published several books and films on these subjects, which are intended both for the expert and the interested general reader.

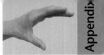

Index